Headache Remedy Guide

Dr. Sheila Harrison

Table of Content

Review

Learn more about the different types of headache, including migraine and tension headache, their symptoms, causes, prevention, home remedies and treatment.

Headaches are a common condition that is characterized by pain that occurs in the head or upper neck area. There are many different types of headaches — common and rare. Here's a guide to 15 recognised types of headaches and how to treat each of them.

Primary Headaches vs. Secondary Headaches

Headaches can be divided into two categories: primary and secondary.

A primary headache occurs as a condition in itself and is not related to any other cause. The main types of primary headaches are migraines, tension headaches, cluster headaches and hypnic headaches.

On the other hand, secondary headaches occur as a result of another condition — this includes hormone headaches that occur due to a change in hormones, head injury headaches that occur after a concussion or whiplash, and even hangover headaches that occur after a night of excessive alcohol consumption.

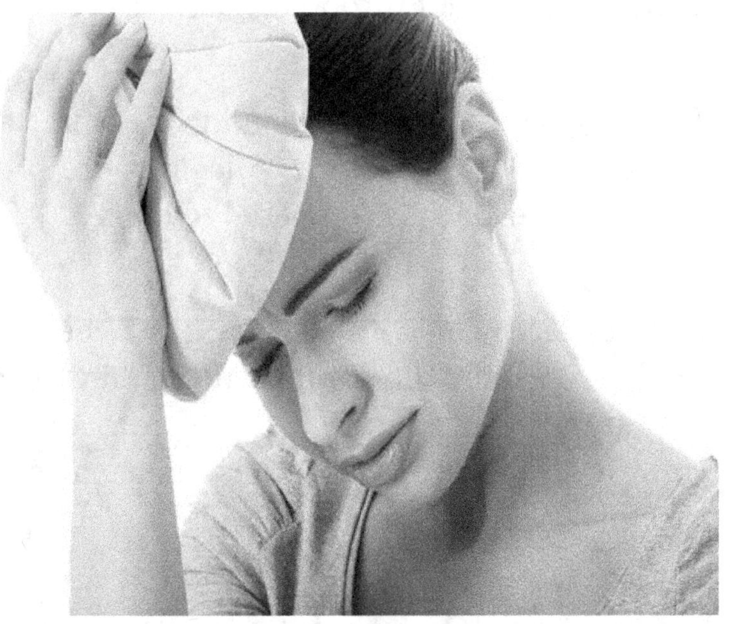

Number 1
Tension Headache

One of the most common types of headaches, tension headaches cause pain behind the eyes and in the base of the neck. Symptoms include muscle tightness in the temple, the sensation of a tight band of pressure around the head, and continuous but not throbbing pain.

The pain can range from mild to severe, and women aged 20 to 40 are typically more prone to tension headaches compared to men.

Most experiences with tension headaches tend to be episodic, meaning that they occur sporadically once or twice a month, or less. However, tension headaches may also be chronic.

Tension headaches are commonly associated with stress, fatigue, arthritis, anxiety or depression, but may also be a result of poor posture, eye strain, as well as misaligned teeth or jawbones.

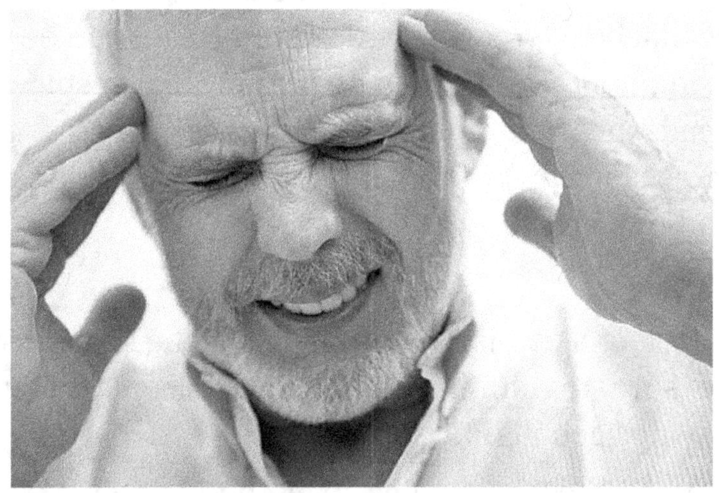

Tension Form of HeadAche

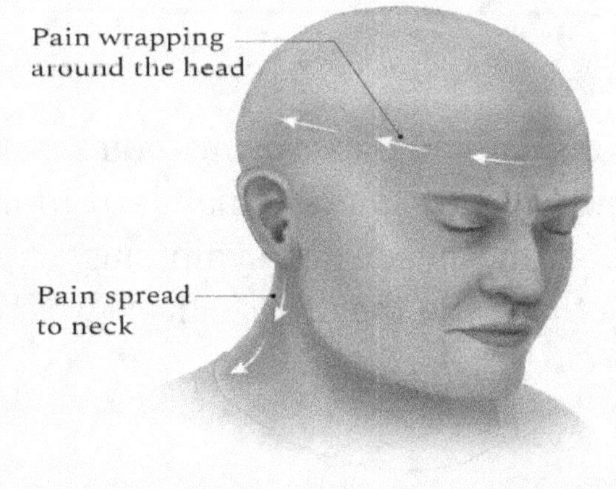

Tension Headache Treatment

When dealing with tension headaches (and most headaches), your first line of treatment can be to drink more water. Dehydration can result in headaches or make headaches worse, so increasing your fluid intake may help mitigate and prevent headaches.

A lack of sleep is a common headache trigger, so be sure to monitor how much sleep you are having each night.

Beyond these strategies, over-the-counter (OTC) medications such as ibuprofen, aspirin and paracetamol may be able to get rid of headache symptoms.

Be cautious about overusing these OTC medications though, as these may lead to more severe recurring headache symptoms as you stop taking them and the drugs' effects wear off.

Number 2
Migraine Headache

Migraines are moderate to severe headaches that manifest as a throbbing pain on one side of the head. This may be accompanied by other symptoms such as feeling nauseous and increased sensitivity to surrounding light and sound.

Migraines are complicated events that may be triggered by different reasons, and the symptoms may manifest differently as well. Though severe chronic migraine attacks can affect one's quality of life, migraines generally occur in a recognisable pattern that makes them easy to diagnose and treat.

What sets a migraine apart from a headache is that it tends to progress through several stages:

1. **The Prodromal Phase**: Pre-migraine warning signs may appear (constipation,

depression, food cravings, hyperactivity, irritability, neck stiffness etc) one to two days before the migraine attack.

2. **The Aura Phase**: Some people may experience visual disturbances or visual auras just before the attack.
Some do not experience this phase, but may instead experience mood changes, fatigue, mental fuzziness, fluid retention, diarrhoea, increased urination, nausea and nasal congestion.

3. **The Attack Phase**: This occurs as a throbbing pain that's usually felt above the eyes and affects one side of the head, which may last for a few hours to several days. Physical activity and movement usually worsen the pain.

4. **The Postdromal Phase**: The pain subsides.

Migraines can happen to anyone, though they tend to be more common in adult women than men. Some women may find that migraine attacks tend to coincide with their menstrual cycle.

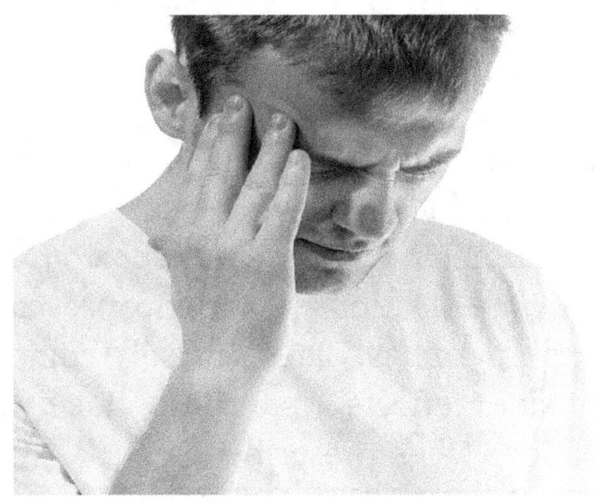

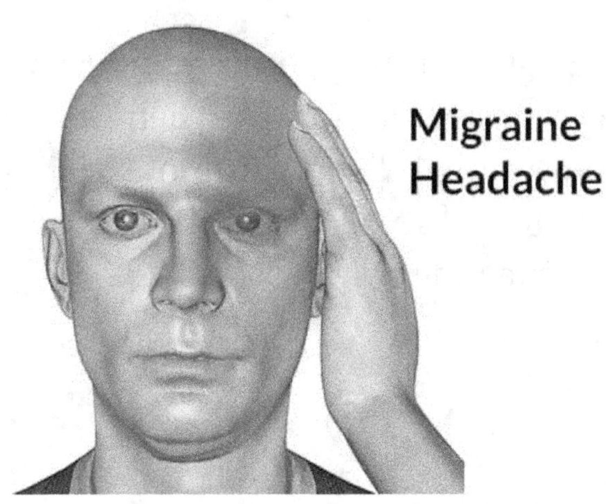

Migraine Headache

Migraine Treatment

Since migraines can be caused by several factors, the best strategy to manage migraines depends on the frequency and severity of your symptoms and how they affect your life.

OTCs such as paracetamol and ibuprofen may help to relieve some migraine pains. However, if your migraines persist, consult a doctor for other treatment options. Some doctors might prescribe medications that help prevent the onset of migraines. These usually come with some side effects, so only take those medications when prescribed.

Staying away from your migraine triggers as much as possible will be helpful. You can consider writing down your potential migraine triggers to help you and your doctor identify them in the long run.

Number 3
Cluster Headache

As its name indicates, cluster headaches are primary headaches that occur in "clusters" of up to eight times per day. This kind of headache can result in severe, debilitating pain that occurs suddenly. This is often considered to be one of the most painful types of headache and is described as a searing, stabbing pain that occurs behind the eye or in the side of the head.

Cluster headaches comprise short attacks that last around 15 minutes to 3 hours. These daily clusters occur in cycles that can last for weeks or months, with cluster headaches occurring daily. Between these cycles is the remission period that can last for months or years, where the individual typically remains headache-free. Those with remission periods that last for less than a month are considered to have chronic cluster headaches.

One key characteristic that separates cluster headaches from migraines is the actions that worsen or lessen the headache's effect during an attack. Migraine patients often opt to lie down in a dark room or keep still during an attack as movement tends to worsen migraines.

On the flip side, most people who suffer from cluster headaches find that keeping still does nothing to help with the pain and tend to fidget and move around during an attack. They may even resort to banging their head on something to distract from the pain.

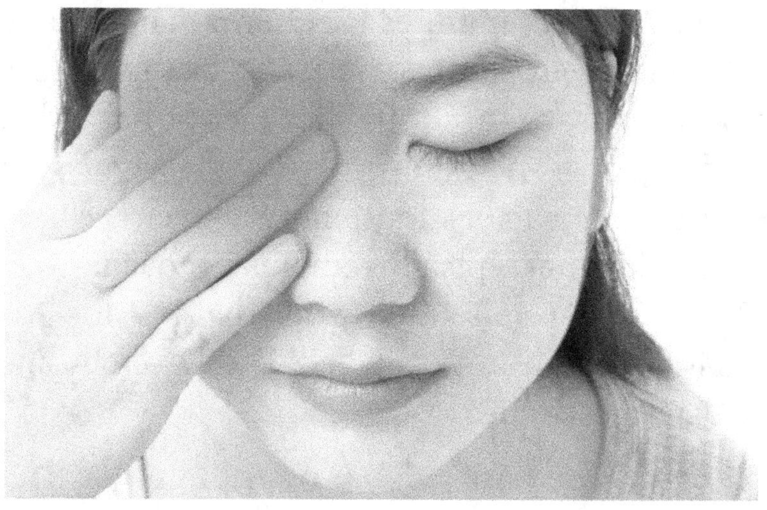

Cluster Headache

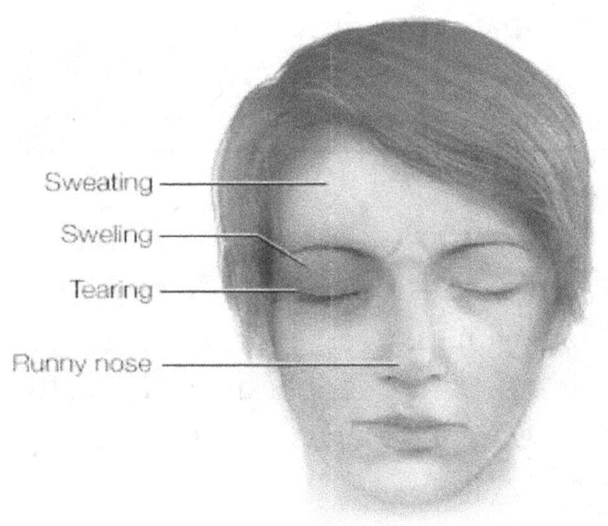

Cluster Headache Treatment

According to the American Migraine Foundation, individuals experiencing cluster headaches are often treated incorrectly by doctors who attempt to treat their symptoms the same way as with migraines. However, cluster headaches and migraines are different forms of headaches that require different types of treatments.

There are several ways that cluster headache symptoms may be reduced, including steroid prescriptions, preventive medications, and other newer experimental treatments that are currently being developed.

The best way to find a treatment plan that works for you is to consult a specialist (neurologist) on an individualised treatment plan for severe headaches that disrupt your quality of life.

Number 4

Hypnic Headache

Hypnic headaches are a rare type of headache that occurs when one is sleeping. These are sometimes called "alarm-clock headaches" for how they awaken people from their sleep.

These headaches often occur around the same time each night for several days a week, with each attack lasting from 15 minutes to 4 hours. The pain can range from mild to severe and may be accompanied by migraine-like symptoms such as nausea as well as light and sound sensitivity.

The exact cause of hypnic headaches is currently still unknown, though some experts believe that they might be linked to issues in the parts of the brain that involve pain management, REM sleep and melatonin production.

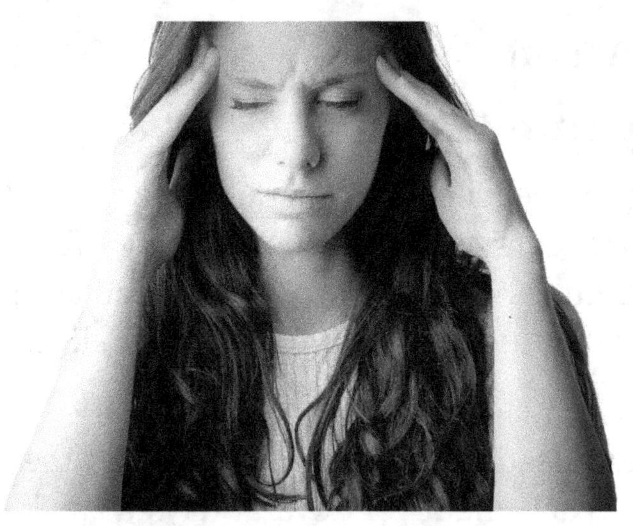

Hypnic Headache Treatment

Though there are currently no specific treatments for hypnic headaches, your doctor might recommend that you try taking a dose of caffeine before bed in the form of coffee, as it has been shown to help reduce hypnic headache attacks without causing any severe side effects.

OTC medications can be taken to manage the pain, though long-term reliance on these may cause chronic headaches. Always speak to your doctor before trying any kind of new medication.

Number 5

Sinus Headache

Sinus headaches (called rhinosinusitis), are a rare secondary headache that occurs due to viral or bacterial sinus infection. Symptoms include thick, discoloured nasal discharge, a decreased sense of smell, facial pain or pressure and fever.

It is quite common for people who "self-diagnose" themselves with sinus headaches to actually be suffering from migraines, due to shared symptoms such as the forehead and facial pressure over the sinuses, nasal congestion and runny nose.

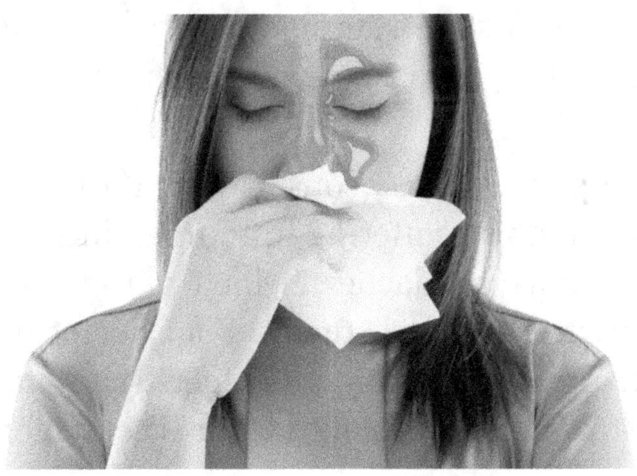

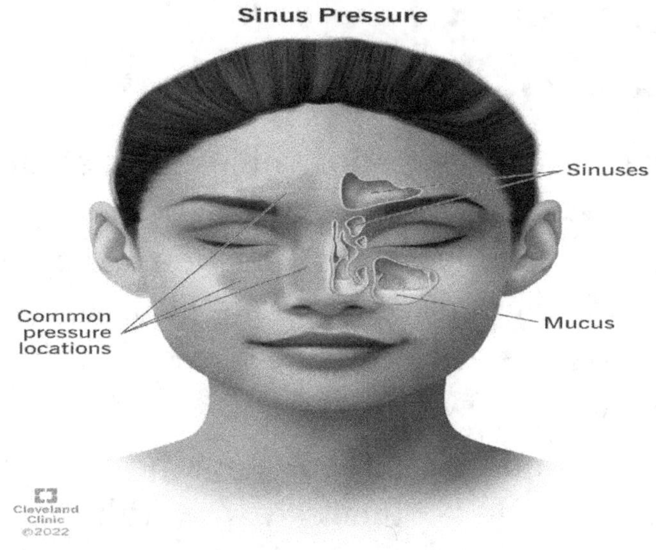

Sinus Headache Treatment

If you have been diagnosed with a bacterial sinus infection, the doctor should prescribe you a course of antibiotics, which should resolve the headache symptoms after a few days.

If the pain persists, consult your doctor again as you may be suffering from migraines rather than sinus headaches, which will require a different type of treatment. Your doctor might then prescribe a migraine-specific treatment for you and see if your symptoms get better.

Number 6

Ocular Migraine

Ocular migraines are a rare condition characterised by temporary vision loss in one eye. This is often caused by reduced blood flow or spasms in blood vessels within the retina or behind the eye.

Ocular migraines can be painless or they can occur along with or after a migraine headache, with vision in the affected eye generally returning to normal within an hour. Symptoms include a small blind spot that affects the central vision in one eye and may get larger, which could end up preventing you from driving or walking if the attack occurs when you are out of the house.

Ocular migraines are often incorrectly used to describe visual migraines, which are much more common and harmless.

Treatment for Ocular Migraine

The first step is to consult your doctor, who will determine if you are suffering from ocular migraines or some other condition. As the attacks usually last less than an hour, most people usually don't require treatment and will be advised to stop their activities during the duration of the attack until their vision returns to normal.

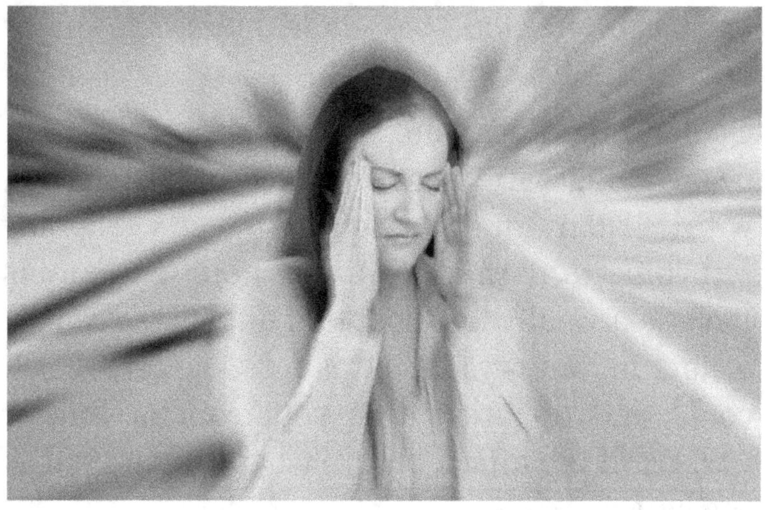

A sudden loss of vision in one eye may be related to a more severe eye problem not linked to headaches. If you suddenly experience any sort of blind spot in your vision, consult an eye doctor immediately to determine if this is a temporary harmless vision problem or a symptom of something more serious such as a retinal detachment or a stroke.

Number 7
Visual Migraine / Migraine Aura

Some people experience a phenomenon called visual migraines or migraine auras shortly before their migraine attack. These often occur suddenly and disappear within 30 minutes or so, and may or may not be accompanied by a migraine headache.

These may manifest as:

1. A flickering blind spot near the centre of one's field of vision

2. A wavy ring of coloured light surrounding a central blind spot

3. A blind spot that slowly migrates across your visual field

One way to determine if you are experiencing an ocular migraine or a visual migraine is to close one eye at a time — if the disturbance occurs in only one eye, it's likely an ocular migraine, and if it occurs in both eyes, it's likely a visual migraine.

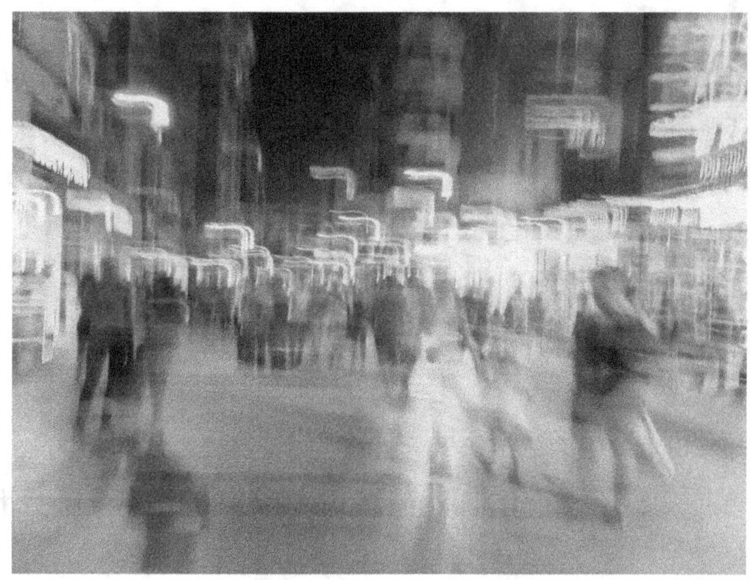

Treatment for Visual Migraine

As with ocular migraines, the first step is to consult a doctor about your vision problems.

The best way to prevent visual migraines is to avoid your migraine triggers and get ample sleep. You may also take OTCs to mitigate the headache pain occasionally.

Number 8

Hormone Headache (Headache During Menstruation)

Due to the natural fluctuations in hormone levels that women experience throughout the month, many women suffer from uncomfortable symptoms around the time of their menstrual cycle, including headaches.

Due to the natural drop in oestrogen levels during this time, migraines are more likely to develop in the two days before a menstrual period or during the first three days of a menstrual period.

Beyond menstrual periods, other causes of hormonal headaches include taking combined oral contraceptive pills (which contain oestrogen) that involve a pill-free week, menopause and pregnancy.

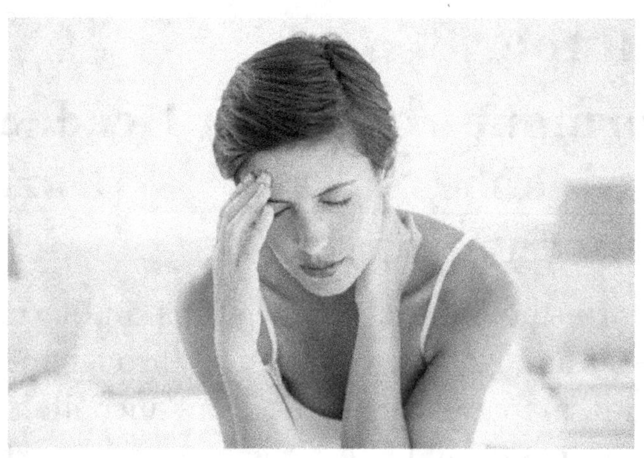

Hormone Headache Treatment

Treatment for hormone headaches typically involves mitigating the headache symptoms via OTCs or prescribed medications taken around the time of one's period.

If your headaches are caused by a drop in oestrogen levels during the pill-free week of taking combined contraceptive pills, you may consult with your doctor on switching to a continuous contraceptive such as combined pills with no break, progesterone-only mini-pills, and birth control implants.

Read our handy guide to learn more about the different types of birth control available in Malaysia.

Number 9
Cervicogenic Headache

A cervicogenic headache is a pain that develops in the neck and radiates to the back and front of the head, often accompanied by neck stiffness. These often result from structural problems in the neck and cervical vertebrae (vertebrae at the top of the spine).

Cervicogenic headaches can develop in people who work in jobs that put them at more risk of neck strain, such as cab drivers and labourers. Cervicogenic headaches can also occur after an injury to the neck such as whiplash.

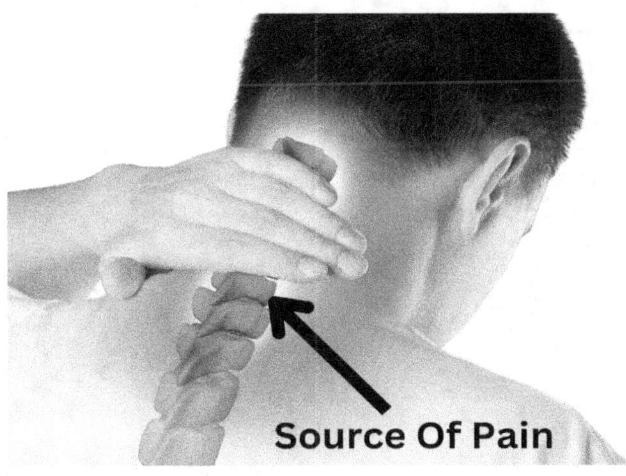

Cervicogenic Headache Treatment

Cervicogenic headache treatment focuses on removing the cause of neck pain. Your doctor may prescribe medication or OTC pain relief medications to help manage the painful symptoms.

Physical therapy involving soft tissue massage and joint movement may also be an effective treatment as it deals directly with the cause of the neck pain that results in cervicogenic headaches.

Number 10

Post-Injury Headache

A post-injury headache is a secondary headache that may occur in the days and weeks following a traumatic head injury.

Headaches immediately after a head injury are fairly common and they usually taper off in the days following it, but a persistent headache that lasts longer than that is considered a post-injury headache.

These types of headaches are often characterised as a daily constant ache that affects both sides of the head. These bouts of pain are usually mild to moderate, though one may experience some spikes in pain similar to that of a migraine.

Other changes and symptoms that people may experience post-injury include neurological symptoms such as dizziness, blurred vision, sleep disruptions and ringing sounds in their ear.

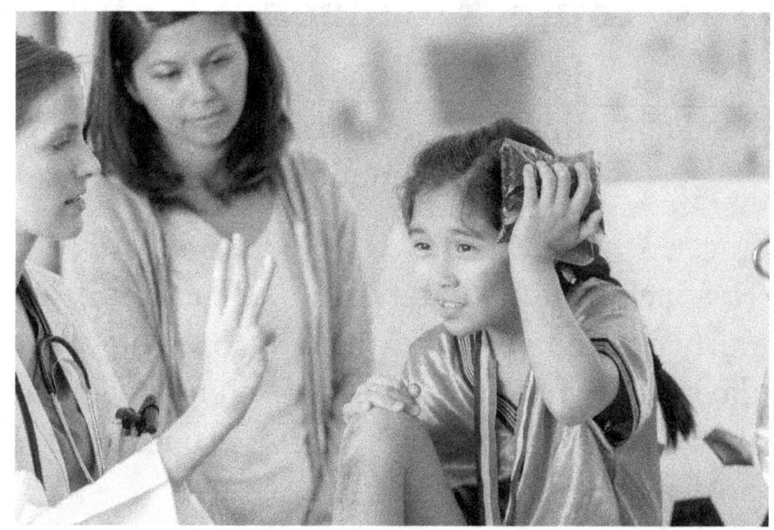

Post-Injury Headache Treatment

Treatment for this type of headache is symptomatic and often consists of tension headache treatments such as medication. Your doctor may also advise you to get ample rest and sleep following a traumatic injury in order to help reduce the symptoms, and to avoid consuming stimulants like nicotine and alcohol.

Number 11
Cough Headache

Cough headaches occur in some people when they experience headaches caused by a bout of coughing that's often triggered by a sudden increase of pressure within the abdomen and chest. These headaches can be either primary or secondary.

If you have sinusitis or a cold, your coughing might become more forceful, which increases your risk of coughing headaches. This headache can also occur after sneezing, laughing, straining during bowel movements and bending over for too long.

These types of headaches are usually nothing serious, particularly if they are primary headaches, which tend to improve on their own. However, secondary coughing headaches could point to a more serious issue (an abnormal skull shape, weakness in a brain blood vessel that could lead to an aneurysm, brain tumour etc).

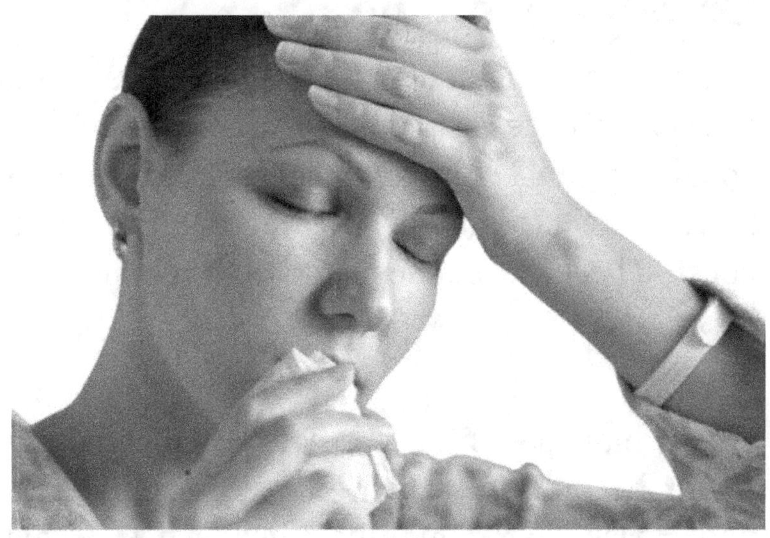

Cough Headache Treatment

Primary cough headaches can often be treated by medication such as OTC anti-inflammatory medications to reduce coughing and blood pressure medication.

Secondary cough headache treatment is more complex and will depend on what the doctor determines the cause to be, whether it's a malformation of the skull or a brain tumour.

Number 12

Exertion Headache (Headache After Exercise)

Exertion headaches are headaches triggered by physical activity such as exercise. This type of headache is often felt as a pulsating pain at both sides of the head during or after a workout, and typically don't last more than several minutes.

Though the causes are unknown, some medical experts believe that strenuous exercise narrows the blood vessels inside the skull and results in headaches. These headaches are often likely to develop when exercising in hot weather or at high altitudes.

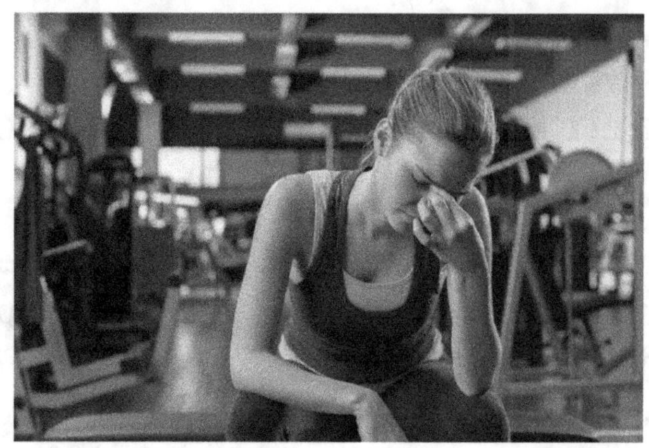

Exertion Headache Treatment

Most exertion headaches go away on their own within a few months. You may take OTC medications to help with the headache pain, as well as apply a hot towel or heating pad to your forehead. You should also drink plenty of fluids before, during, and after exercise to prevent dehydration.

If you frequently get headaches after exercising and experience other unusual symptoms, make an appointment with your doctor to rule out any serious underlying conditions.

Number 13
Stimulant Drug Headache

Headaches and migraines are associated with individuals with attention deficit disorder (ADD) and attention deficit hyperactivity disorder (ADHD) who are prescribed stimulant drug medication, such as Adderall.

Most individuals report two different types of headaches when using medications to treat ADHD and ADD. The first is a milder sort of headache that is usually felt at the back of the head, which occurs at the end of the dose. This type of headache is relatively bearable and can usually be relieved by taking OTCs if desired.

The second type of headache tends to be more severe and is usually felt radiating throughout the whole head for the entire duration of the dose (and sometimes even after each dose has worn off). Patients with a family history of migraines are often more susceptible to this type of severe headache side effects.

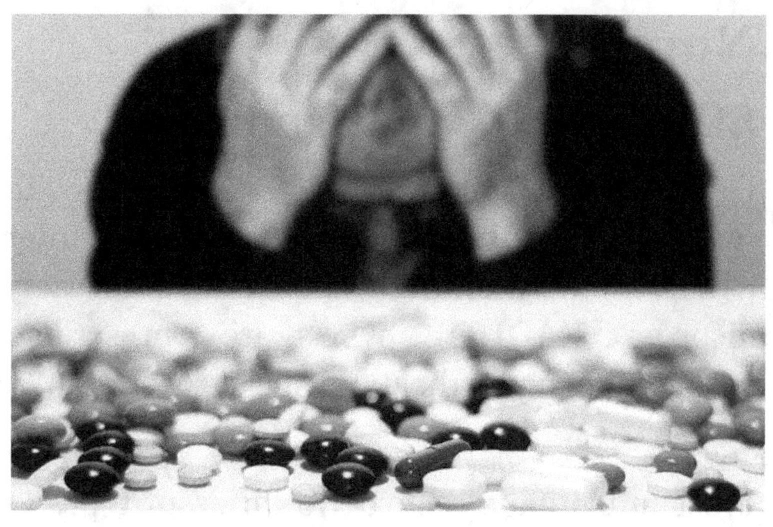

Stimulant Drug Headache Treatment

If you experience recurring headaches as a side effect of your prescription, consult your doctor for the best course of treatment. Your doctor might consider switching the type of medication prescribed to help with the symptoms.

Number 14

Caffeine Headache

Did you know that caffeine can both cause and relieve headaches?

Headaches can be caused by a caffeine overdose. Caffeine isn't just found in coffee — it's found in energy drinks, workout supplements such as pre-workout, certain sodas as well as other foods and beverages. One side-effect of caffeine is that it makes you urinate more (as it is a diuretic), which is dehydrating. In turn, dehydration can cause headaches.

On the flip side, caffeine can also help treat headaches. Some people are prescribed caffeine by their doctor in a bid to alleviate chronic headaches — particularly patients with hypnic headaches.

However, once your body adapts to caffeine, stopping consumption for even one day could cause some unpleasant side effects. Since caffeine narrows the blood vessels that surround the brain, a sudden stop in consumption results in these blood vessels dilating. The increase in blood flow around the brain puts pressure on the surrounding nerves, which may trigger caffeine withdrawal headaches.

This can happen to anyone who consumes coffee regularly, even in doses as little as a cup of coffee a day. If you've been taking caffeine to alleviate your headaches, stopping the consumption of caffeine may result in a "rebound effect" during which your headaches become worse after you stop — similar to how an overreliance on medication for headaches can result in a worse headache after you stop taking it.

Caffeine Headache Treatment

There is no actual way to prevent or stop caffeine headaches from occurring. However, if you consume caffeine regularly, you can monitor your intake to ensure that you are not taking too much caffeine each day. Drink plenty of water as well to make sure that your body is well-hydrated since caffeine is a diuretic.

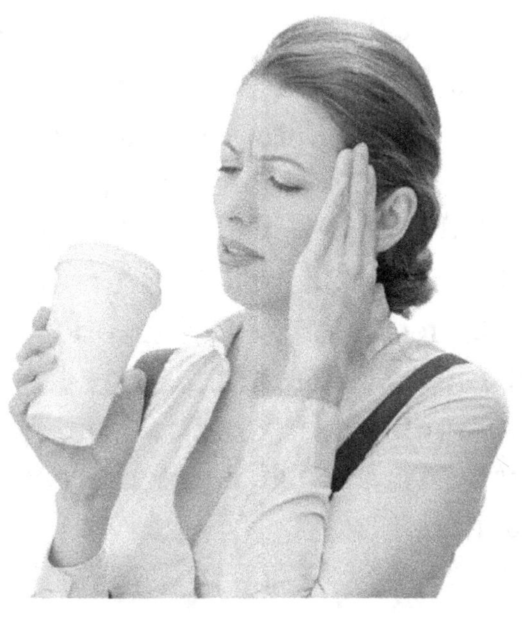

Number 15
Hangover Headache

Wine nights are great for unwinding — but having a few too many glasses may result in some unpleasant morning afters.

Despite how warm and fuzzy alcohol often makes you feel, it's still a substance that affects your brain, liver, kidneys and other body systems adversely. Many of these effects persist till the next day even after your body detoxes from the alcohol. Dehydration is one significant effect, alongside disruptions to your blood chemistry, digestion, and sleep cycle. These all cumulate in what we come to know as the hangover, which is often accompanied by headaches.

The duration of each hangover varies depending on how much alcohol was consumed, how hydrated (or dehydrated) you are, weight, gender, current health status and more. People who are already prone to migraines tend to experience more instances of developing headaches along with their hangovers.

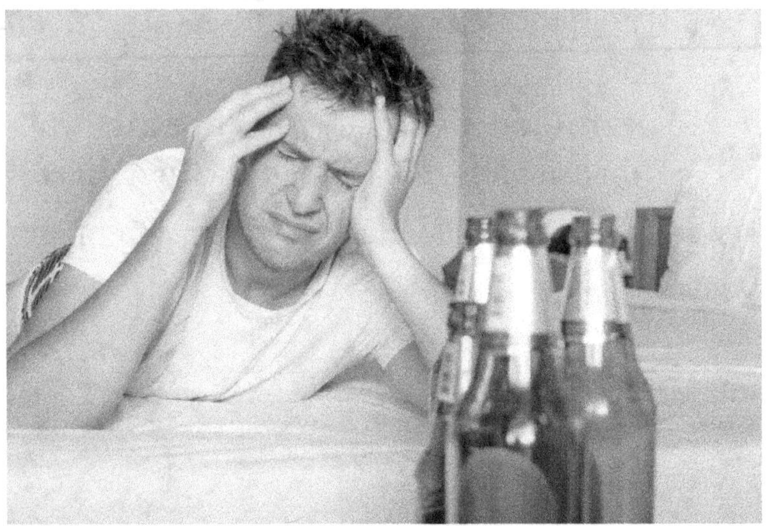

Hangover Headache Treatment

Despite all the hangover drinks and jellies that claim to prevent hangovers, the best and most reliable way to avoid a hangover is: don't drink.

If you end up with a splitting headache after a night of overindulgence, here are some things you can do:

- Drink more fluids (other than alcohol) to stave off dehydration, such as water and sports drinks.

- Don't take medications like acetaminophen that may overtax your liver (and definitely don't drink when you are on medication in the first place)

- Avoid more alcohol — that's a given.

When to See a Doctor for Headaches?

Most headaches are usually mild and will go away with rest and the occasional self-medication. If your headache is chronic, you may want to consult a GP or be referred to a specialist who can devise a treatment plan for you.

Even though most headaches don't require immediate medical intervention, persistent and severe headaches may point to more serious problems that require immediate medical attention.

Consult a doctor immediately or head to the emergency department if your headache:

- Is abrupt and severe, and/or lasts over 72 hours with little to no gaps
- Occurs with a fever
- Happens after a head injury and gets worse
- Lasts for a few days or weeks and gets worse after coughing, exertion, straining or a sudden movement

- Is accompanied by severe and uncontrollable vomiting
- Occurs along with confusion and difficulty in understanding what other people are saying

www.ingramcontent.com/pod-product-compliance
Lightning Source LLC
Chambersburg PA
CBHW070742260726
48660CB00007B/2948